GET RID OF YOUR BUTT

TIGHTER BUNS, THINNER THIGHS IN 75 MINUTES A WEEK

BY JEANETTE MICELOTTA, M.S., P.T.,
AND DEBORAH MICHAELS, P.T.A.
WITH MARILYN J. APPLEBERG

INTRODUCTION BY DR. RICHARD BACHRACH

DIRECTOR, CENTER FOR SPORTS AND OSTEOPATHIC MEDICINE

PHOTOGRAPHY BY ELLEN WALLOP

A JOHN BOSWELL ASSOCIATES BOOK
HEARST BOOKS
NEW YORK

Library of Congress Cataloging-in-Publication Data
Micelotta, Jeanette.
     Get rid of your butt / Jeanette Micelotta and Deborah Michaels.
        p.   cm.
     ISBN 0-688-12982-X
     1. Reducing exercises.   2. Buttocks.   I. Michaels, Deborah.   II. Title.
    RA781.6.M53   1994
    613.7'1—dc20   93-6405
                                                          CIP

Printed in the United States of America
First Edition

1 2 3 4 5 6 7 8 9 10

BOOK DESIGN BY Barbara Cohen Aronica
Models: Michael T. Brown
       Claudia Porfilio

Contents

Introduction
By Richard Bachrach, D.O.

At the Center for Sports and Osteopathic Medicine I see patients of both sexes, of every age and occupation. I treat bankers, corporate executives, dentists, lawyers, writers, actors, accountants, and even physicians. Typically, what they do best and most is sit. Sitting, however, can be dangerous. The more we sit, the bigger and softer becomes that on which we sit. Man or woman, bottom-heavy not only looks terrible, it can be painful—because a portly posterior can put too much stress on the lower back.

Through a combination of buttock and abdominal muscle strengthening, we help relieve and prevent the recurrence of low back pain in such patients. With improved fitness and strength, posture improves. Patients are easily able to translate the benefits of the exercise program into improved performance of everyday activities such as walking, standing, sitting, carrying, and lifting. They are amazed by their newfound increase in energy and ease of movement. Perhaps most significantly, they feel better about themselves. By following the program presented in this book, you can easily reap the harvest of what they had to learn the hard way.

Get Rid of Your Butt was written by Jeanette Micelotta and Deborah Michaels, the same outstanding therapists from the Center for Sports and Osteopathic Medicine who created *Get Rid of Your Gut*. As noted in their first book, progress may appear to be dreadfully slow. Don't be discouraged! Generally, older people and those beginning a program at a relatively high level of fitness will respond more slowly. Be patient, and, *stay with it*. The beneficial effects of exercise are quickly reversible. Make a regular exercise program a way of life.

1

Get Rid of Your Butt: The 75-Minute Solution

Nearly everyone agrees that a toned, well-proportioned silhouette is pleasing to the eye. When you look at yourself in the mirror—either dressed or undressed—is that what you see reflected? Or does a droopy bottom keep you from seeing your ideal? Well, you are not alone, and there are solid reasons why the posteriors of both men and women are often less than perfect.

Unlike the abdominal muscles, which are in constant use and are therefore continuously "exercised" in the normal course of the day, the main muscle of the buttock region—the gluteus maximus—is totally underutilized. It doesn't do any work—it just sits there.

Indeed, for most of the population, sitting is an occupational hazard. Not only on the job, but at home, and in between in cars, buses, or trains, we tend to spend a great many hours sitting. The end result of all this sitting for most people is that their bottom is often not the tops.

But even if you have been a self-described couch potato, you need not resign yourself to being forever bottom-heavy. The solution is simple—all you have to do is resolve to do something about it and

1

then follow through. Buying this book was a good first step in that direction.

The good news is that the muscles of the gluteal region can and do respond to exercise, and the program we have developed is designed to lift, trim, firm, tone, and generally improve the appearance of your presently less-than-perfect posterior. By sticking to the regimen we have worked out, you will begin to see some results in as little as one month. Your butt will appear smaller due to the toning.

In addition you will find that proper execution of all of the exercises in the program require you to use your stomach muscles consciously to hold the normal curve of the spine. Learning the all-important abdominal contraction (see page 12) will not only help you get the most out of your buttock workout, it will also result in a flatter, stronger abdomen.

The exercises presented in this book are not only designed to tone and strengthen the buttock muscles, they also strengthen the lower back. This is particularly true of the bridge, the squat, and the lunge. Each of these exercises, in which the feet are stationary and fixed and the body is moving, uses several muscle groups at once, requiring you to employ both your back and abdominals to stabilize your trunk. Doing these results in increased balance, coordination, and stability.

The exercises in which the foot is free and moving through space (the posterior leg raise, buttock kick, bilateral prone hip extension, side leg raise, and rotation) focus specifically on the gluteal region. They also work the lower back, particularly in the advanced level where trunk stability is required for the standing positions. The beginner and intermediate phases of the program use exercises that require much less coordination but they focus totally on the muscle group you want to work—the glutes.

As you learn more about this region of the body, and how important it is in maintaining a strong and flexible torso, the easier it will be for you to make these exercises a part of your normal routine. You will find the benefits of this program so numerous that with a minimum of 75 minutes a week, a strong, toned, and well-formed buttocks is the least of what you will achieve.

VIVE LA DIFFERENCE

The exercises in this book are designed to be done by and to benefit both sexes. But because there are differences between men and women in fat distribution and levels of strength, the results may be markedly different.

Men tend to have larger muscles, so strengthening the gluteal muscles may be a lot easier for a man (the abdomen, of course, is another matter). Also, the larger a muscle, the more force it can generate, and because men generally develop larger muscles, their strength is proportionally greater than that of a woman. Since women by nature are endowed with more body fat than men (5–6 percent more), they tend to be loaded down with more of what might best be described as "dead" weight. It's also an unfortunate fact that in addition to what nature endowed her with, any excess weight a woman gains in her lifetime will generally take up residence around her hips, so achieving the derriere of her dreams may take a little longer. Any woman who wants to pare down her posterior significantly *must* combine the exercise program with a reduced fat diet and aerobic exercise. Yet we can state unequivocally that for both sexes who undertake our Classic Buttock Program—and stick with it—the results will soon be obvious in how you look and how you feel.

BEGINNING A FITNESS PROGRAM

It is imperative before starting any fitness program to consult your doctor to ascertain that you are in good general health or if there should be any restrictions on the duration or intensity of your workouts. Anyone beginning an exercise program should start slowly, gradually building strength and flexibility while carefully monitoring his or her progress.

INJURY PREVENTION

One should incorporate *all* phases of a proper training program in order to maximize the benefits and minimize the possibility of injury. We recommend the following injury-prevention steps to be done in this specific order:

The warm-up prepares the muscles, ligaments, and tendons for action. It steps up blood circulation, raises body temperature, and enhances flexibility of the joints. By limbering the muscles and joints, these exercises can prevent many injuries. The warm-up should consist of either some calisthenics, biking, running in place, or light resistance exercise. Each body part should be moved through a full range of motion. A warm-up of at least 5 minutes of any rhythmic-type movement is a must to encourage blood flow into the muscles and prepare them for more strenuous activity. Once the warm-up is completed you should be perspiring lightly and be ready to begin the training program.

Stretching is done following the warm-up and before the training program to prepare the muscles for the necessary flexibility for sports or a training program. Stretching *must* be done after the training program as a cool down.

The training program includes setting goals, such as the number of days of training, where the training will be done, and at what time of day. It also includes executing the proper form of exercises as well as your nutrition, diet, and the amount of rest you require.

The cool down should be done after completing the entire exercise routine. It helps the body make the transition from high-intensity activity to a normal level, encouraging muscles that have been strongly contracted to relax and become more stretched and flexible. Low-grade calisthenics, a light jog, biking, and the like are useful for cooling down. Stretching is an absolute must at this time and can help to prevent muscle soreness.

THE GLUTEALS: A QUICK PRIMER

THE MUSCLES OF THE GLUTEAL REGION

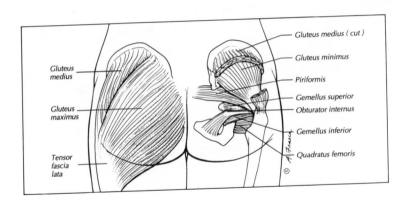

The buttock area is made up of one very large muscle, the *gluteus maximus,* and many smaller muscles underlying it, the most important of which are the *piriformis, tensor fascia lata,* and the *gluteus medius* and *minimus.* These muscles begin in the pelvis and end in the upper part of the thigh bone. Their principal functions are to turn the thigh outward, and to extend it to the back and/or to the side. More important, they act with the abdominals and hamstrings in stabilizing the pelvis, counteracting the hip flexors, and maintaining good postural alignment.

STRONG ABS, BACK, AND GLUTES

It would be nice if we could just work on the one area of our body we perceive as less than perfect—the butt—and not think about the rest of our muscles, but it can't be done. As the song says, the knee bone *is* connected to the shin bone and in doing exercises to firm and tone the butt, your abdominal and back muscles are brought into play in a big way. You cannot properly execute the exercises in the program without making moves that will simultaneously utilize and strengthen the abdominal and back muscles.

The trunk is the body's center of power. This is true not only in the context of athletic activities but with all of our everyday activities, whether bending, carrying, or lifting. That's why a balanced exercise program is one that strengthens all of the trunk muscles—the abs, the back, *and* the glutes—and in the process corrects bad posture, which can lead to back pain, preventing you from correctly performing not only exercise but everyday tasks.

The abdominal muscles—*rectus abdominis* and the *internal* and *external obliques*—are part of the group that forms the trunk musculature. Weak abdominals are a primary cause of bad posture and may be a predisposing factor in chronic lower back pain. Strong and flexible back muscles are also essential for maintaining good posture as well as allowing for an unrestricted range of motion. Strengthening these muscles can reduce the risk of injuries that may occur from everyday activities.

The buttocks—*gluteus maximus*—is the most important extensor muscle controlling the lower back's lifting power and, together with the abdominals, they provide stability to the spine. The simultaneous contraction of all of these muscles, particularly the obliques, provides a corseting effect for the lower spine.

In accordance with the most recent research, our buttock exercise program has been designed to achieve a balance of abdominal, buttock, and back extensor strength, in order to deal adequately with the stress forces placed on the spine on a daily basis.

2

Getting Started:
What You Need to Know

THE EXERCISES

Posterior Leg Raise
Buttock Kick
Rotation
Side Leg Raise

Bilateral Prone Hip Extension
Bridge
Squat
Lunge

DO IT RIGHT!

It is important for you to know from the start that in order to perform correctly the exercises that make up the Classic Buttock Exercises, you will have to learn the abdominal contraction. As we stated in the previous chapter, you cannot isolate your butt from your gut; in order to strengthen and tone the buttock you must simultaneously contract your abdomen as well as your back extensors. That is why we have included learning the abdominal contraction as part of your preparation for embarking on our program.

You should also be aware of the fact that bad form can sabotage your progress, leaving you with zero results or worse. Doing exercises correctly minimizes your risk of injury and maximizes your exercise efforts. Mastering the abdominal contraction will help provide the trunk stability necessary to maintaining proper form during execution of each of the above moves, and as an added bonus it will help strengthen and tone your abs. To help ensure proper form, be certain to follow all of the pointers accompanying each of the exercises.

GET THE MOST OUT OF THE PROGRAM

The type of training program we have designed is one that uses sets and reps, with three different levels of intensity—beginner, intermediate, and advanced. You will find that the sets and reps vary a bit as each level comes closer to the next more difficult and challenging one. Each rep should be performed slowly enough to enable you to concentrate on form and technique. Maintaining this control will allow you to get the most out of each of the exercises. We recommend that the entire buttock-strengthening regime be done 3–4 times weekly. For best results, the exercises should be done in the sequence described in the program designed for each level. Training sessions are constructed to last 20 minutes, including the essential rest stops, plus the essential 5 minutes of stretching outlined in chapter 4.

YOUR TRAINING LEVEL

The following should help you find the specific exercise level to suit your abilities. If you are in doubt, be conservative and choose one that may be beneath your abilities. You can easily move to the next level if you find you need more of a challenge.

BEGINNER LEVEL

If you are in poor physical condition, have never exercised, or have exercised less than twice a week for the past 2–3 months, or if you are overweight, start at the beginner level and perform 1 set of 10 repetitions of each exercise indicated in this level of the program. Once you become stronger and find that the increasing reps and sets have become easier, it's time to go on to the intermediate level for more of a challenge.

INTERMEDIATE LEVEL

If you have graduated from the beginner level or if you already exercise with some regularity and find the beginner level too easy but the advanced too strenuous, then the intermediate level is for you.

Start at this level with 2 sets of 10 repetitions and then move through the program doing the increasing reps and sets of the exercises indicated. When you reach the point where this is no longer taxing your muscles, you are ready to move to the advanced level.

ADVANCED LEVEL

If you have graduated from the intermediate level, or are already in great physical shape, with strong buttock muscles and abdominals, start at this level. Start by performing 2 sets of 10 reps of the prescribed exercises, moving to a maximum of 4 sets of 12 reps.

REPS AND SETS

A rep, or repetition, is the number of times you perform the same exercise of a set from start to finish. A set is a number of reps performed without stopping for a rest. As you get stronger, you increase the number of reps and sets per exercise. For beginners, we have found that performing 10 repetitions of each exercise for 3 sets by the second week of the program is the best way to build strength and achieve tone.

REST BETWEEN SETS

You should allow 30 seconds of rest time between sets to give your working muscles adequate time to recuperate after you have pushed them. If you skip or decrease the resting time, the more taxed your muscles and heart may feel, and the less energy you may have to continue. Ultimately, skipping the 30 seconds of rest may lead you to curtail your workout, or worse, it may result in an overuse injury.

A FULL DAY OF REST

There are rest days scheduled in the program but if you find yourself particularly tired or pressed for time, take an extra day off from the aerobic and upper body or abdominal part of the program. Try to be consistent in the 3-4-times-weekly buttocks workout plan.

BREATHING

The most important thing to know about breathing during all strength training is that you inhale just *before* you start the exertion phase of the movement and then exhale slowly on the exertion. You inhale through the nose and exhale through pursed lips. *Never* hold your breath between repetitions of an exercise. Holding your breath during exercise could impede the flow of blood to the arteries of the heart, and you could become light-headed or could faint.

MUSCLE SORENESS

When starting an exercise program or resuming a program following an extended layoff, you may experience muscle soreness. This soreness should not discourage you from continuing to exercise; on the contrary, more exercise is the best remedy. Soreness may persist for several hours immediately after exercise, but it generally appears later and may last for 3–4 days.

Two types of soreness can result from muscle strain: acute and delayed. Acute muscle soreness is often caused by inadequate blood flow to the muscles; the 30- to 60-second rest period between each *set* in weighted exercise helps prevent this type of soreness. Delayed muscle soreness is thought to result from eccentric or muscle-lengthening exercise only. This form of soreness is commonly noticed between 24 and 48 hours after exercise. If the soreness doesn't lessen or completely disappear within a few days or if you begin to feel any sharp pains, stop the exercises and check with your doctor.

WHEN TO EXERCISE

In order to ensure consistency in your conditioning program, exercises should be done when most convenient for you. It is important to note that first thing in the morning may not be the best time for you to engage in physical fitness. At that time the discs in the back are less resilient, the joints are stiffer, and the muscles are less flexible. But if morning is the only time you are able to do the program, be cognizant of the aforementioned and be extra diligent in your stretching exercises to compensate for the stiffness and lack of flexibility.

Exercising in the early evening may be more natural. Exercise causes a rise in body temperature, leading to a feeling of mental alertness. That's why you may start your workout feeling tired after a day's work but will end up feeling energized and ready for an evening out. After 5 or 6 hours, your temperature drops and you will feel tired once again. Therefore, the best workout time might be just before dinner, so the subsequent drop in body temperature will coincide with your normal bedtime.

There is an added benefit to exercising about an hour before dinner.

Working out has an effect on the hypothalamus—the part of the brain that controls hunger—causing a reduction in appetite at precisely the right time. The only don'ts to remember when trying to establish an exercise habit is to avoid exercising just before bed or immediately after meals.

THE ALL-IMPORTANT ABDOMINAL CONTRACTION

As we stated before, learning the abdominal contraction is an important element in proper performance of the buttock program outlined in chapter 3. The contraction is an isometric exercise unto itself, so not only will you be toning your butt, you will also be toning your gut.

Begin by inhaling deeply through your nose. As you exhale, the natural tendency is to let your abdominal muscles go limp. You must consciously fight this tendency by tensing the abdominal muscles. Anatomically, the idea is to lower the ribs down toward the belly button while simultaneously lifting the pubic (groin) bone up toward the belly button. You should also maintain a slight arch in your back. The abdominal contraction is not as complicated as it may sound. In order to feel the results you are seeking, cough a couple of times; the tightening of the abdominal muscles just as you cough approximates the sensation you want to achieve. You should also feel the isometric pressure against the rib cage and the groin area from this contraction. You must remember to inhale deeply when your body is at rest, then exhale and contract simultaneously as you lean into the exercise.

Once this contraction is learned, it should be utilized not just for buttock exercises, but during sitting, standing, and walking throughout the day. As a result, you will be strengthening your abdominals every time you make a conscious effort to contract them.

3

The Classic
Buttock Exercises

There are several things to keep in mind as you begin this program. First, we cannot emphasize enough that all of these exercises require a simultaneous contraction of the abdominals and back extensors, in order to provide the trunk stability and proper form that is essential during the workout. Also, since you will probably perform these exercises on your own, in your home, how successful you will be depends completely on you. Be conscious of your body and what it tells you, both at the beginning and end of your workout. If you are feeling overly tired you may be doing too much too soon; don't go beyond your capabilities by overestimating your fitness level or rushing to the next phase. Learn to listen to your body; soreness, not pain, is normal. Remember, too, as was discussed in chapter 2, the ache you feel upon embarking on an exercise regime is normal, will be relieved by more exercise (soreness is not an excuse to stop), and should disappear in just a few days.

THE EXERCISES

Note once again that all of these exercises require a simultaneous contraction of the abdominals and back extensors to provide the trunk stability necessary for proper execution. Also keep in mind that pelvic positioning is key to postural control of the lower back. In addition, adequate flexibility of the hamstrings, quads, psoas, calf muscles, and hip rotators is important for natural, pain-free movement. All of these are used and strengthened with our program. We recommend that the entire program be performed at least 4 times a week.

SPECIFIC (OPEN CHAIN) EXERCISES

Posterior Leg Raise: buttock (*gluteus maximus*), hamstring, back extensors

Buttock Kick: buttock (*gluteus maximus*), back extensors

Rotation: internal (*gluteus minimus, tensor fascia lata, gluteus medius*) and external (*obturators, gemellis, piriformis, quadratus femoris, gluteus maximus*) rotators

Side Leg Raise: *gluteus medius* and *gluteus minimus*

Bilateral Prone Hip Extension: *gluteus maximus,* hamstrings, back extensors

FUNCTIONAL (CLOSED CHAIN) EXERCISES

Bridge

Squat

Lunge

The exercises above use multiple muscle groups including buttocks (*gluteus maximus*), hamstrings, quads, calves, abs, and back extensors. In the execution of each, the *gluteus medius* and *gluteus minimus* act as pelvic stabilizers.

Strengthening for the Gluteals
1. Posterior Leg Raise

Beginner Level

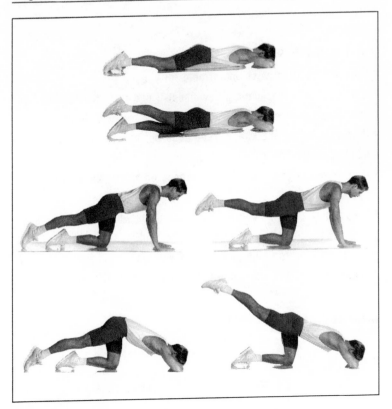

FORM
- Lie on your stomach, or hands and knees, or forearms and knees.
- If using alternative position to stomach, extend right leg out behind you, foot relaxed with toes resting on floor; pelvis is level.

EXECUTION
- Tighten stomach using abdominal contraction; keep trunk straight, maintaining normal curve.

- Inhale.
- Exhale and slowly lift right leg up from the hip until leg is in line with the trunk.
- Inhale and slowly return to start.
- Repeat the sequence until all sets are completed.
- Switch to left leg and repeat.

POINTERS
- Choose a position most comfortable for you.
- If on your stomach, use a pillow under it and rest your forehead on your hands.
- If on your hands and knees, keep head in line with trunk, with hands directly under the shoulders and knees hip-width apart.
- If on forearms and knees, rest forehead on hands, knees hip-width apart.
- Keep pelvis straight; don't allow it to roll outward on exercising leg or allow the pelvis to drop on the supported leg.
- Don't raise leg too high or your back will arch.
- Keep buttock tight, particularly during execution of exercise.

Intermediate Level

FORM
As in beginner level. (Choose 1 of 3 positions on page 15.)

EXECUTION
- Tighten stomach using abdominal contraction; keep trunk straight, maintaining normal curve.
- Inhale.
- Exhale and slowly lift right leg up from hip until leg is in line with trunk.
- Once leg is elevated, breathe normally and perform small pulses until set is complete; only then will you return to start.

- Repeat the sequence until all sets are completed.
- Switch to left leg and repeat.

POINTERS
As in beginner level.

Advanced Level

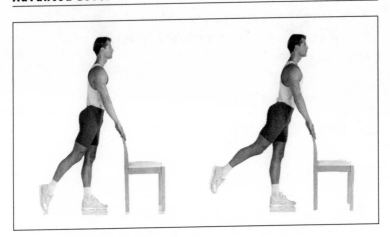

FORM
- Stand and gently hold onto wall or back of chair (for balance only).
- Trunk is straight but leaning slightly forward from hips, head is in line with trunk, eyes level, feet parallel and slightly apart, pelvis level and facing forward.
- Extend right leg out behind you, foot relaxed and toes resting on floor.

EXECUTION
- Tighten stomach using abdominal contraction; keep trunk straight, maintaining normal curve.
- Breathe normally.
- Lift right leg up from hip only far enough so as not to arch low

back (this motion may be as slight as toes only 3 inches off the floor).
- Keep buttock tight and perform pulses until set is complete, then return to start.
- Repeat the sequence until all sets are completed.
- Switch to left leg and repeat.

POINTERS
- Don't lift leg so high that lower back arches.
- Don't allow pelvis to rotate toward the extended leg.
- Don't lock standing leg.

2. Buttock Kick

Beginner Level

FORM
- Lie on stomach, or hands and knees, or forearms and knees.
- If on stomach, bend knee to 90 degrees.

EXECUTION
- Tighten stomach using abdominal contraction; keep trunk straight, maintaining normal curve.
- Inhale.
- Exhale and slowly lift right leg up from hip until thigh is in line with trunk.
- Inhale and slowly return to start with thighs parallel.
- Repeat the sequence until all sets are completed.
- Switch to left leg and repeat.

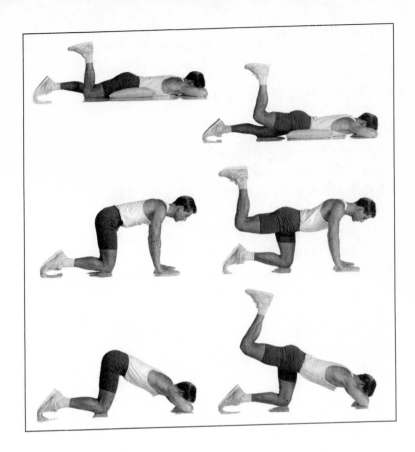

POINTERS

- Choose a position most comfortable for you.
- If on your stomach, use a pillow under it and rest forehead on hands.
- If on hands and knees, keep head in line with trunk, hands directly under shoulders and knees hip-width apart.
- If on forearms and knees, rest forehead on hands; keep knees hip-width apart.
- Don't allow pelvis to roll outward on exercising leg or drop on supported leg.
- Don't raise leg too high or your back will arch.
- Tighten buttock particularly during execution of exercise.

Intermediate Level

FORM
As in beginner level. (Choose 1 of 3 positions on page 19.)

EXECUTION
- Tighten stomach using abdominal contraction; keep trunk straight, maintaining normal curve.
- Breathe normally and slowly lift right leg from the hip until leg is in line with the trunk.
- Once leg is elevated, perform small pulses until set is complete, then return to start.
- Repeat the sequence until all sets are completed.
- Switch to left leg and repeat.

POINTERS
As in beginner level.

3. Rotation

Beginner Level

FORM
- Lie on your right side with hips and knees bent to a 45-degree angle, resting head on hand, hips facing forward, trunk straight, head and feet relaxed.
- Free arm is in front of you with hand on floor for balance.

EXECUTION
- Tighten stomach using abdominal contraction; keep trunk straight, maintaining normal curve.
- Inhale.

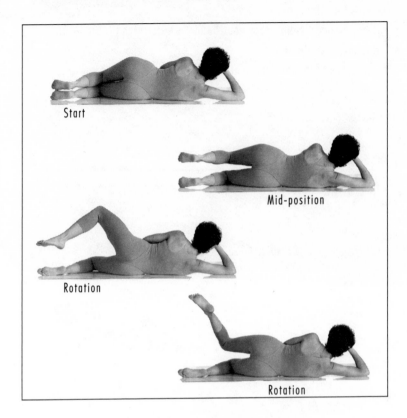

Start

Mid-position

Rotation

Rotation

- Maintaining the leg angles, lift left leg up from hip (midposition).
- Exhale and slowly rotate leg upward from hip until knee is pointing toward the ceiling and the top foot is over the bottom foot.
- Inhale and return to midposition.
- Exhale and slowly rotate leg downward until knee is pointing toward bottom knee and top thigh is over bottom thigh.
- Inhale and return to midposition, then to starting position.
- Repeat the sequence until all sets are completed.
- Switch to left side and repeat.

POINTERS
- Keep trunk straight and don't allow low back to arch.
- Don't allow pelvis to rock forward or backward with leg motions.

- If more comfortable, rest your head on outstretched arm or on forearm and elbow.
- If you are able, repeat several rotations before returning to start.

Intermediate Level

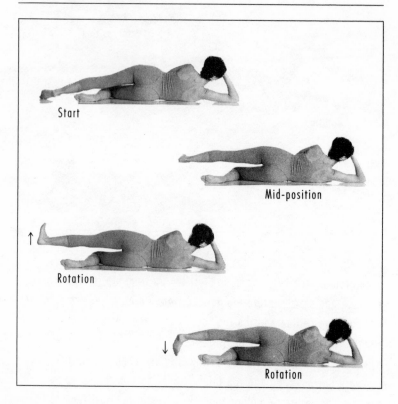

Start

Mid-position

↑ Rotation

↓ Rotation

FORM
- Lie on your right side, resting head on hand, hips facing forward, trunk straight and head and feet relaxed.
- Bend bottom hip and knee to 45-degree angle with left leg straight out in line with trunk, knee facing straight ahead.
- Free arm is in front of you with hand on floor for balance.

EXECUTION

- Tighten stomach using abdominal contraction; keep trunk straight, maintaining normal curve.
- Inhale and slowly raise the leg from hip until parallel to the floor (midposition).
- Exhale and, continuing to breathe normally, rotate the leg in small pulses so that knee is alternately directed toward the ceiling and then toward the floor. The movements of these rotations are minimal.
- Continue performing the pulses until set is complete and only then return to start.
- Repeat the sequence until all sets are completed.
- Switch to left side and repeat.

POINTERS

- Keep trunk straight and don't allow low back to arch.
- Don't allow pelvis to rock forward or backward with leg motions.
- Don't allow leg to move forward or backward from line of trunk.
- Don't allow knee to lock.
- Don't raise the leg higher than parallel.
- If more comfortable, rest your head on outstretched arm or lean on forearm and elbow.

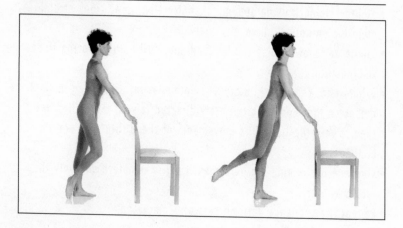

FORM

- Stand and gently hold on to wall or back of chair for balance only.
- Keep trunk straight but leaning slightly forward from hips, head in line with trunk, eyes level, pelvis level, and facing forward.
- Right foot is relaxed, toes resting on floor and even with left heel, knee bent and rotated outward.

EXECUTION

- Tighten stomach using abdominal contraction; keep trunk straight, maintaining normal curve.
- Breath normally and, maintaining position, lift right leg up from hip only far enough so as not to arch low back (this motion may be as slight as toes 3–4 inches off floor).
- Keep buttock tight and perform pulses until set is complete and only then return to start.
- Repeat the sequence until all sets are completed.
- Switch to left leg and repeat.

- Don't lift leg so high that lower back arches.
- Don't allow pelvis to rotate toward the extended leg.
- Don't lock standing leg.

4. Side Leg Raise

Beginner Level Only

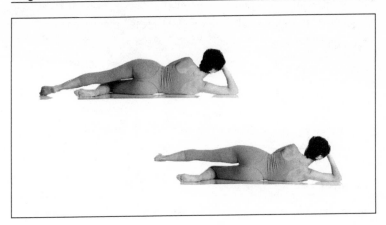

FORM

- Lie on your right side resting head on hand, hips facing forward, trunk straight, and head and feet relaxed.
- Bend bottom hip and knee to 45-degree angle with left leg straight out in line with trunk, knee facing straight ahead.
- Free arm is in front of you with hand on floor for balance.

EXECUTION

- Tighten stomach using abdominal contraction; keep trunk straight, maintaining normal curve.
- Inhale.
- Exhale and slowly raise leg from hip until it is parallel to the floor.

- Inhale and slowly return to start.
- Repeat the sequence until all sets are completed.
- Switch to left side and repeat.

POINTERS
- Keep trunk straight and don't allow low back to arch.
- Don't allow pelvis to rock forward or backward with leg motions.
- Don't allow leg to move forward or backward from line of trunk.
- Don't allow knee to lock.
- Don't raise the leg higher than parallel.
- If more comfortable, rest head on outstretched arm or lean on forearm and elbow.

5. Bridge

Beginner Level

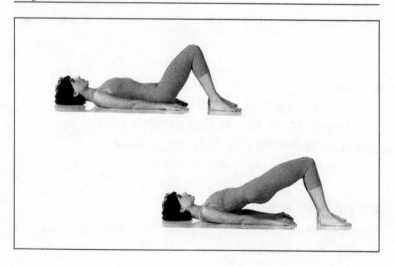

FORM

- Lie on your back with your arms at your sides, knees bent, and feet flat on floor, turned slightly outward and hip-width apart.
- Head and neck are relaxed.

EXECUTION

- Tighten stomach using abdominal contraction; keep trunk straight, maintaining normal curve.
- Inhale.
- Keeping stomach and buttock tight, exhale and slowly lift buttock off floor by pushing down on feet.
- Allow head, shoulders, and shoulder blades to remain on floor.
- Inhale and slowly return to start.
- Repeat until all sets are completed.

POINTERS

- Don't allow buttock to raise so high that lower back arches and abdominal contraction is lost.
- Don't use hands to help raise buttock.
- Distribute weight equally on both feet.
- Make a special effort to push feet into floor with each lift.
- Keep pelvis level.

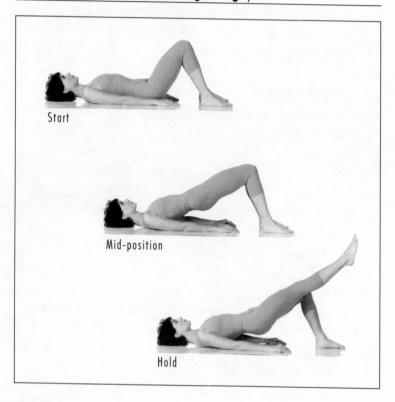

Start

Mid-position

Hold

FORM

As in beginner level.

EXECUTION

- Tighten stomach using abdominal contraction; keep trunk straight, maintaining normal curve.
- Inhale.
- Keeping stomach and buttock tight, exhale and slowly lift buttock up off the floor by pushing down on feet.
- Allow head, shoulders, and shoulder blades to remain on floor.
- Slowly straighten knee of right leg, keeping in line with thigh of supporting leg, foot relaxed, knee facing the ceiling.

- Hold for 5 seconds.
- Inhale and slowly return to start by first bringing foot back to the floor, then lowering buttock to the floor.
- Repeat sequence until all sets are completed.
- Switch to left leg and repeat.

POINTERS

- Don't allow buttock to raise so high that lower back arches and abdominal contraction is lost.
- Don't use hands to help raise buttock.
- Distribute weight equally on both feet.
- Make a special effort to push supporting foot into floor with each lift.
- Don't allow pelvis to drop, especially on unsupported side.
- Don't allow elevated leg to rotate in or out.

Advanced Level

FORM
As in beginner and intermediate levels.

EXECUTION
- Tighten stomach using abdominal contraction; keep trunk straight, maintaining normal curve.
- Inhale.
- Keeping stomach and buttock tight, exhale and slowly lift buttock up off the floor by pushing down on feet.
- Allow head, shoulders, and shoulder blades to remain on floor.
- Slowly straighten knee of right leg, keeping in line with thigh of supporting leg, foot relaxed, and knee facing ceiling.
- Breathing normally while maintaining this position and pushing

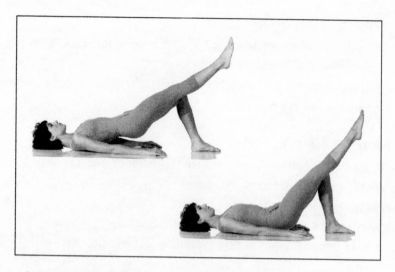

down onto supporting foot, with buttocks tightened, perform small
pulses, raising and lowering pelvis only 2–3 inches.
- Continue performing the pulses until the set is complete.
- Inhale and slowly return to start by first bringing foot back to the
  floor, followed by lowering buttock to the floor.
- Repeat the sequence until all sets are completed.
- Switch to left leg and repeat.

POINTERS
As in intermediate level.

6. Squat

Beginner Level–Quarter Squat

FORM
- Stand with arms at your side, head relaxed and in line with trunk,
  eyes straight ahead, knees relaxed, feet turned slightly outward
  and shoulder-width apart.

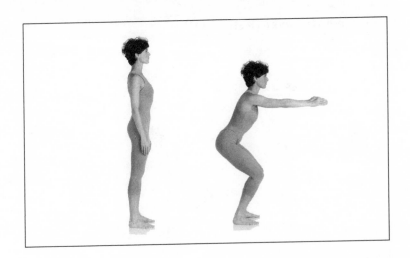

EXECUTION

- Tighten stomach using abdominal contraction; keep trunk straight, maintaining normal curve.
- Inhale.
- Exhale and slowly bend hips and knees to approximately a 45-degree angle by leaning trunk forward and extending buttock out behind you, keeping heels on floor.
- Simultaneously raise arms up in front of you to shoulder level.
- Inhale and return to the starting position by emphasizing the push of your feet into the floor, tightening your buttock, straightening your legs, and lowering your arms.
- Repeat sequence until all sets are completed.

POINTERS

- Keep head in line with trunk throughout the execution of the exercise.
- Keep back straight and don't allow lower back to arch excessively.
- Keep knees centered over feet at all times, don't allow them to move ahead of toes.
- If your calves are tight, either raise up on the toes or put something under the heels.

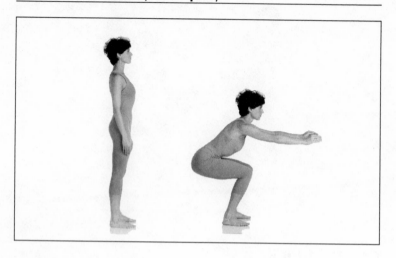

FORM
As in beginner level.

EXECUTION
- Tighten stomach using abdominal contraction; keep trunk straight, maintaining normal curve.
- Inhale.
- Exhale and slowly bend hips and knees to approximately a 90-degree angle (with thighs parallel to floor) by leaning trunk forward and extending buttock behind you, keeping heels on floor.
- Inhale and return to starting position by emphasizing the push of your feet into the floor, tightening your buttock, and straightening your legs.
- Repeat sequence until all sets are completed.

POINTERS
As in beginner level.

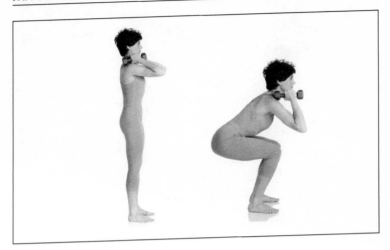

FORM

- Stand with your arms at your sides, head relaxed and in line with trunk, eyes straight ahead, knees relaxed, feet turned slightly outward and shoulder-width apart.
- Lift two 5-pound dumbbells to your shoulders; elbows are in line with shoulders and pointing straight ahead.

EXECUTION

- Tighten stomach using abdominal contraction; keep trunk straight, maintaining normal curve.
- Inhale.
- Exhale and slowly bend hips and knees to approximately a 90-degree angle by leaning trunk forward and extending buttock out behind you, keeping heels on floor.
- Inhale and return to starting position by emphasizing the push of your feet into the floor, tightening your buttock and straightening your legs.
- Repeat the sequence until all sets are completed.

POINTERS
- As in beginner level.
- Reduce size of weight if execution is difficult or proper position is difficult to maintain.

7. Forward Lunge

Intermediate Level

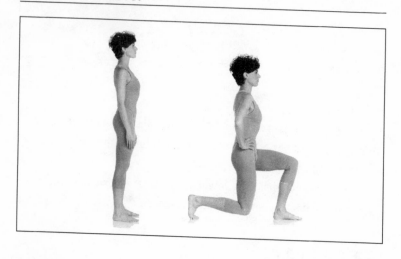

FORM
- Stand with arms at your sides or hands on hips, head relaxed and in line with trunk, eyes straight ahead, knees relaxed, feet turned slightly outward and hip-width apart.

EXECUTION
- Tighten stomach using abdominal contraction; keep trunk straight, maintaining normal curve.
- Inhale.
- Exhale and slowly step forward with the left leg leading with the heel so that both knees bend to approximately a 90-degree angle

34

(left thigh is parallel to the floor, right thigh is perpendicular to the floor).
- Inhale and return to starting position by emphasizing the push of the feet into the floor, with buttock tightening as legs are straightening and left leg moves back.
- Repeat sequence until all sets are completed.
- Switch to right leg and repeat.

POINTERS
- Keep head in line with trunk throughout the execution of the exercise.
- Keep back straight and don't allow lower back to arch.
- Keep knees centered over feet at all times.
- Don't allow knees to move ahead of toes (step far enough forward).
- Don't allow trunk to move forward or backward.

Alternative Lunge: Backward Lunge

Intermediate Level

This exercise can be used as an alternative to the forward lunge. You may find it easier to maintain proper form during the execution.

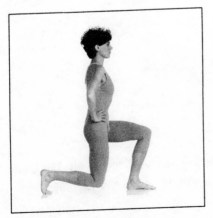

FORM
As in forward lunge.

EXECUTION

- Tighten stomach using abdominal contraction; keep trunk straight, maintaining normal curve.
- Inhale.
- Exhale and slowly step backward with the right leg leading with the toe, so that both knees bend to a 90-degree angle (right thigh perpendicular to the floor and left thigh parallel to the floor).
- Inhale and return to starting position by emphasizing the push of the feet into the floor, with buttock tightening as legs are straightening and right leg moves forward.
- Repeat sequence until all sets are completed.
- Switch to left leg.

POINTERS

As in forward lunge.

Advanced Level

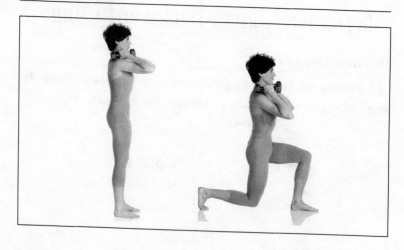

FORM

- As in intermediate level, except 2-5-pound dumbbells are held on the shoulders, elbows in line with shoulders and pointing straight ahead.

EXECUTION

As in intermediate forward/backward lunge.

POINTERS

As in intermediate forward/backward lunge.

8. Bilateral Prone Hip Extensions

Advanced Level Only

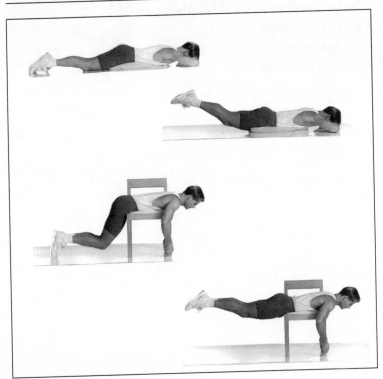

POSITION

• Lie on your stomach with forehead resting on hand and pillow under stomach or standing and leaning trunk over bench, chair, table, or the like, bending at the hips, head in line with trunk.

EXECUTION

- Tighten stomach using abdominal contraction; keep trunk straight, maintaining normal curve.
- Inhale.
- Exhale and slowly lift both legs up from the hips, keeping knees straight until legs are in line with the trunk.
- Inhale and return to start.
- Repeat sequence until all sets are completed.

POINTERS

- Choose a position most comfortable for you.
- Keep pelvis straight.
- Don't raise legs so high that lower back arches.
- Tighten buttock particularly during execution of exercise.

4

The Program

Beyond the difficulty most people have in overcoming inertia and starting an exercise program, and after the initial burst of commitment and the feeling of achievement and exhilaration, the next difficulty comes in sticking with it. As we mentioned earlier, finding the best time to perform these exercises is a personal choice. *When* you do them is not important; what is paramount is *that* you do them. The benefits of an exercise regime are soon lost if you stop doing it, and before long you are back to where you started.

Though starting and sticking with a program requires discipline, so do most things with high rewards. Brushing your teeth, for example, is such an ingrained habit that you wouldn't think of leaving the house without doing it. Well, exercise is just as important—if not more so —to your total health and appearance. That's also the reason behind doing the program at the same time of day and in the same part of the house or apartment every time—it helps to establish routine. After doing these exercises for several weeks, performing them will become habitual. Then, when you start to see and feel the difference in your body, it will become more difficult to skip them than to do them. You'll soon find that exercise is one habit you won't want to break.

GENERAL PROGRAM GUIDELINES

The exercise program recommended here assumes three distinct levels of fitness and progresses from one to the next as your muscles get stronger. See pages 8–9 to determine which level you should begin with, depending on your own fitness level. It is best not to do too much too soon, since you might be risking muscle fatigue or worse. The three levels of the exercise program are described below.

Beginner level. For the first 13 days of the program this level incorporates 4 exercises—posterior leg raise, buttock kick, rotation, and side leg raise (program exercises 1–4)—then adds the bridge and squat (exercises 5 and 6), and gradually increases in both repetitions and sets. Exercising at this low-intensity level allows the body to adapt safely, comfortably, and progressively to the stresses and demands each of the different exercises places on your muscles. You may stay at this entry level as long as you like. Note that exercise 4 is in the beginner level only, since the leg raise is incorporated into the intermediate rotation. In weeks 3 and 4 you are actually in transition to the intermediate level.

Intermediate level. This level, which also incorporates exercises 1–6, uses a higher level of intensity and in exercises 1 and 2 changes the lifts to pulses, movements of very small range of motion that occur at or near maximum contraction of the muscle. The exercise position is held throughout and these small movements are performed without returning to the start position, maintaining an isometric type of contraction. Not resting between reps makes this a more difficult workout. Exercises 3 and 4 are combined in this level, 5 and 6 increase in difficulty, in week 6 Day 13, program exercise 7, the lunge is introduced.

Advanced level. At this level, in weeks 9 and 10, you will be executing only 5 exercises: advanced hip extension and advanced rotation, bridge, squat, and forward or backward lunge (exercises 1, 3, 5, 6, 7); after a day of rest, on the twelfth day of week 10, you add the more difficult advanced levels of the bridge, squat, and lunge (exercises 5, 6, 7), as well as 1 set of 12 reps of the newly introduced bilateral prone hip extension, program exercise 8. At this level all exercises may increase to the maximum, 4 sets of 12 reps, as feasible. The standing positions of the advanced exercise level require even more tightening of stomach muscles with a simultaneous contraction of back extensors to prevent the lower back from arching and to stay balanced, stable, and properly aligned. At this level the *gluteus medius* and the *gluteus minimus* (the muscles used in the side leg raise, exercise 4) are used to stabilize the pelvis, keeping the proper alignment.

THE TWELVE WEEKS

The following sample chart is set up in 4-week increments, each progressing but generally reflecting a beginning, intermediate, and advanced level of fitness.

MONTH 1

BEGINNER LEVEL
Beginner Exercises   1. posterior leg raise; 2. buttock kick; 3. rotation; 4. side leg raise; 5. bridge; 6. quarter squat

Beginner Program   Weeks 1 and 2, exercises 1–4; add exercises 5 and 6 on day 6 of week 2

W E E K 1

Day 1   Exercises 1–4: 1 set of 10 reps
Day 2   Same

Day 3	Rest
Day 4	Exercises 1–4: 1 set of 12 reps
Day 5	Rest
Day 6	Exercises 1–4: 1 set of 12 reps
Day 7	Rest

WEEK 2

Day 8	Exercises 1-4: 2 sets of 10 reps
Day 9	Same
Day 10	Rest
Day 11	Exercises 1–4: 2 sets of 12 reps
Day 12	Rest
Day 13	Exercises 1–4: 3 sets of 10 reps
	Exercises 5 and 6: 1 set of 10 reps
Day 14	Rest

Beginner/Intermediate Program   Weeks 3 and 4, exercises 1–6

This is a transitional phase to enable you to acclimate slowly to the newly introduced exercises, beginning with low reps and sets and then increasing both per the program.

WEEK 3

Day 15	Exercises 1–4: 3 sets of 10 reps
	Exercises 5 and 6: 1 set of 10 reps
Day 16	Same
Day 17	Rest
Day 18	Exercises 1–4: 3 sets of 12 reps
	Exercises 5 and 6: 1 set of 12 reps
Day 19	Rest
Day 20	Exercises 1–4: 4 sets of 10 reps
	Exercises 5 and 6: 1 set of 12 reps
Day 21	Rest

WEEK 4

Day 22	Exercises 1–4: 4 sets of 10 reps
	Exercises 5 and 6: 2 sets of 10 reps
Day 23	Same
Day 24	Rest
Day 25	Exercises 1–4: 4 sets of 12 reps
	Exercises 5 and 6: 2 sets of 12 reps
Day 26	Rest
Day 27	Exercises 1–4: 4 sets of 12 reps
	Exercises 5 and 6: 2 sets of 12 reps
Day 28	Rest

MONTH 2

INTERMEDIATE LEVEL

Intermediate Exercises 1. posterior leg raise with pulses; 2. buttock kick with pulses; 3.–4. combine into intermediate exercise 3, side leg raise with pulses and rotations; 5. bridge with leg raise; 6. half squats; 7. lunge

Intermediate Program Weeks 5 and 6 will introduce new intermediate exercises 1–3 but will continue with exercises 5 and 6 at the Beginner/Intermediate Level. Day 13 of week 6, change to intermediate-level exercises 5 and 6 and the new exercise, the lunge. Weeks 7 and 8, intermediate exercises 1–7 as described above.

WEEK 5

Day 1	Exercises 1–3: 2 sets of 10 reps
	Beginner/Intermediate exercises 5 and 6: 2 sets of 12 reps
Day 2	Same
Day 3	Rest
Day 4	Exercises 1–3: 2 sets of 12 reps
	Beginner/Intermediate exercises 5 and 6: 2 sets of 12 reps

Day 5   Rest
Day 6   Exercises 1–3: 3 sets of 10 reps
        Beginner/Intermediate exercises 5 and 6: 3 sets of 10 reps
Day 7   Rest

WEEK 6

Day 8   Exercises 1–3: 3 sets of 10 reps
        Beginner/Intermediate exercises 5 and 6: 3 sets of 10 reps
Day 9   Same
Day 10 Rest
Day 11 Exercises 1–3: 3 sets of 12 reps
        Beginner/Intermediate exercises 5 and 6: 3 sets of 12 reps
Day 12 Rest
Day 13 Exercises 1–3: 4 sets of 10 reps
        Intermediate-level exercises 5 and 6: 1 set of 10 reps
        Exercise 7: 1 set of 10 reps
Day 14 Rest

Intermediate/Advanced Program   Weeks 7 and 8
Intermediate Exercises 1–7

WEEK 7

Day 15 Exercises 1–3: 4 sets of 10 reps
        Exercises 5–7: 1 set of 10 reps
Day 16 Same
Day 17 Rest
Day 18 Exercises 1–3: 4 sets of 12 reps
        Exercises 5–7: 1 set of 12 reps
Day 19 Rest
Day 20 Exercises 1–3: 4 sets of 12 reps
        Exercises 5–7: 1 set of 12 reps
Day 21 Rest

WEEK 8

Day 21 Exercises 1–3: 4 sets of 12 reps
               Exercises 5-7: 2 sets of 10 reps

Day 22 Same

Day 23 Rest

Day 24 Exercises 1–3: 4 sets of 12 reps
               Exercises 5–7: 2 sets of 12 reps

Day 25 Rest

Day 26 Exercises 1–3: 4 sets of 12 reps
               Exercises 5-7: 2 sets of 12 reps

Day 27 Rest

MONTH 3

ADVANCED LEVEL

Advanced Exercises 1. standing hip extension; 2. intermediate 2, 3 combine into advanced exercise 3, advanced hip rotation; 5. bridge with pulses; 6. half squat with weights; 7. lunge with weights. Also new exercise, 8, bilateral hip extension is added.
* Note: Intermediate exercise 4 (side leg raise) has been incorporated into the standing exercises.

Advanced Program Weeks 9 and 10 will introduce advanced exercises 1 and 2, but will continue with exercises 5–7 on the Intermediate/Advanced Level. Weeks 11 and 12, advanced exercises 1–8 as described above.

WEEK 9

Day 1 Exercises 1 and 3: 2 sets of 10 reps
          Intermediate/Advanced exercises 5–7: 2 sets of 12 reps

Day 2 Rest

Day 3 Exercises 1 and 3: 2 sets of 12 reps
          Intermediate/Advanced exercises 5–7: 2 sets of 12 reps

Day 4	Rest
Day 5	Exercises 1 and 3: 2 sets of 12 reps
	Intermediate/Advanced exercises 5–7: 2 sets of 12 reps
Day 6	Rest
Day 7	Rest

W E E K 10

Day 8	Exercises 1 and 3: 3 sets of 10 reps
	Intermediate/Advanced exercises 5–7: 3 sets of 10 reps
Day 9	Rest
Day 10	Exercises 1 and 3: 3 sets of 10 reps
	Intermediate/Advanced exercises 5–7: 3 sets of 10 reps
Day 11	Rest
Day 12	Exercises 1 and 3: 3 sets of 12 reps
	Advanced-level exercises 5–7: 1 set of 12 reps
	Exercise 8: 1 set of 12 reps
Day 13	Rest
Day 14	Rest

Advanced/Advanced Program   Weeks 11 and 12
Advanced Exercises 1, 3, 5, 6, 7, 8

W E E K 11

Day 15	Exercises 1 and 3: 4 sets of 10 reps
	Exercises 5–8: 1 set of 12 reps
Day 16	Rest
Day 17	Exercises 1 and 3: 4 sets of 12 reps
	Exercises 5–8: 1 set of 12 reps
Day 18	Rest
Day 19	Exercises 1 and 3: 4 sets of 12 reps
	Exercises 5–8: 2 sets of 10 reps
Day 20	Rest
Day 21	Rest

Day 22	Exercises 1 and 3: 4 sets of 12 reps
	Exercises 5–8: 2 sets of 10 reps
Day 23	Rest
Day 24	Exercises 1 and 3: 4 sets of 12 reps
	Exercises 5–8: 2 sets of 12 reps
Day 25	Rest
Day 26	Exercises 1 and 3: 4 sets of 12 reps
	Exercises 5–8: 2 sets of 12 reps
Day 27	Rest
Day 28	Rest

At this level all exercises may increase to the maximum, 4 sets of 12 reps as feasible.

INCORPORATING THE BUTTOCK EXERCISE PROGRAM INTO A GENERAL CONDITIONING PROGRAM

While our exercise program will strengthen and tone your buttock muscles, we recommend that it be incorporated into a general conditioning program of aerobic exercise as well as upper-body and abdominal workout for more total fitness, better general muscle tone, and injury prevention. Be sure to do a warm-up before beginning workouts. Aerobic exercises such as bicycling, walking, or light jogging are great for getting the blood circulating. An upper-body workout can consist of push-ups and dips. The classic buttock program takes care of the lower body; for abs see *Get Rid of Your Gut.* The stretching program presented in chapter 5 should keep you limber.

WEEKLY GENERAL CONDITIONING PROGRAM

Day 1   Aerobics (biking, walking, jogging—20 minutes)
Lower body (15 minutes)
Abdominals (16 minutes)
Stretching (5–7 minutes)

Day 2   Upper body (push-ups and dips, 5 minutes)
Abdominals
Stretching

Day 3   Aerobics
Lower body
Stretching

Day 4   Upper body
Abdominals
Stretching
If lower body exercises are being done 4 times weekly, add them here

Day 5   Rest; however, stretching should be done this day

Day 6   Aerobics
Lower body
Abdominals
Stretching

Day 7   Aerobics
Upper body
Stretching

P R O G R A M   G U I D E L I N E S

- Lower body and upper body exercises alternate days to allow for full recovery.
- Abdominal workouts are scheduled 4 days a week; they are an integral part of the lower-body workout.
- The program provides for 4 weekly aerobics workouts, each lasting at least 20 minutes.

- There is one full day of rest scheduled to give your body an opportunity to recover fully from the demands of the program.
- Stretching should be done every day, including on your rest day.

AEROBIC TRAINING AND DIET

Note that aerobics are a necessary added ingredient to this program, especially if fat reduction and weight loss are goals. Aerobic or endurance exercise utilizes oxygen to break down sources of energy in the body. This is generally prolonged exercise lasting at least 20–30 minutes. Aerobic exercise affects and improves heart and respiratory rates *if* the exercise is performed at a sufficient intensity to increase the heart rate to about 70 percent of its maximum.

Maximum heart rate is age-dependent and can easily be calculated by subtracting your age from 220. Training at 60 to 80 percent of this number (depending upon your physical condition) will effectively condition the aerobic system. Take the example of a healthy 50-year-old: $220 - 50 = 170$; 70 percent of $170 = 119$, which is the pulse rate he or she should achieve for best results.

Ideally, aerobic exercise should be done at least 3–4 times per week. These exercises should involve large muscle groups activated in a rhythmic nature such as in biking, walking, running, stair climbing, skating, or swimming. Performing one or more of these activities for at least 20 minutes several times during the week is all that it takes to achieve and sustain significant health benefits.

To determine fitness for this type of activity, a physical exam should be done for adults over age 35 prior to engaging in aerobic workouts. For everyone, regardless of fitness level, training should begin at a relatively moderate intensity and gradually lead up to the target level. Several minutes of a warm-up, so that heart and circulation are not suddenly taxed, are done first and a five-minute cool down, consisting of exercise gradually lessening in intensity, is generally recommended before the aerobic exercise is stopped. We recommend following this regime in order to reduce the chances of abrupt changes in the cardiovascular system.

5

The 5-Minute Stretch

As with all exercise it is imperative that stretching exercises be performed correctly. The exercise should focus on the range of motion of a particular muscle group and stretch only far enough to feel tension—not pain. Note that muscles need to be relaxed in order to stretch further, because overstretching activates the protective stretch mechanism called the stretch reflex. This nerve reflex sends a signal to the muscle to contract rather than stretch, producing an involuntary contraction that keeps the muscle from being injured or overstretched.

Any strenuous exercising should be followed by *at least* 5 minutes of a slow, passive stretching program. It is useful in preventing injury, particularly with certain muscle groups that tend to become too tight with repetitive use and it is *essential* in exercise programs such as this one which focus on a particular muscle group. Stretching should be done slowly and gently without bouncing—*never* bounce. The position should be comfortable and held for at least 20 seconds. There should be no strain, no pain, no holding of breath.

THE STRETCHING ROUTINE

The following stretches are specifically designed to stretch the buttock muscles, the low back muscles, and the hips, thighs, and calves. It should take you between 5 and 7 minutes to perform all of the stretches presented in this chapter.

Low Back Stretch on Heels

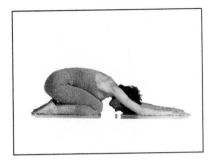

F O R M
- On your hands and knees, head in line with trunk, hands shoulder-width apart, hips and knees at 90-degree angles, knees hip-width apart.

E X E C U T I O N
- Begin slowly moving buttock back onto your heels (your upper body should be rounded).
- Arms are outstretched as far as possible in front of you.
- Rest forehead on the floor.
- Relax and hold for 20 seconds.

Stretch is felt along back and buttock.

Lying Buttock/Hip Stretch

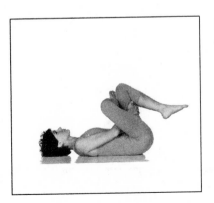

F O R M
- On your back with knees bent, feet flat on the floor.
- Cross your right ankle over the left thigh and bring your legs toward your chest.
- Intertwine fingers behind left thigh just below the knee.

EXECUTION

- To stretch right buttock gently pull left knee toward your chest and hold for 20 seconds.
- Return to start and repeat with left leg.

Stretch is felt in buttock on each side.

Low Back Stretch

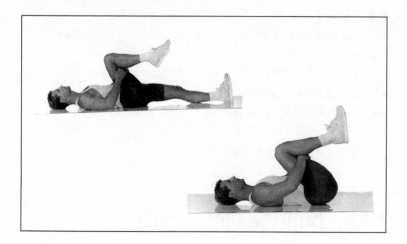

Alternate knee to chest and both knees to chest.

FORM

- On your back with knees bent, feet flat on the floor.

EXECUTION (knee to chest)

- Gently pull right knee toward your chest with your hands around your thigh as you extend the opposite leg out and onto the floor.
- Keep abdominals contracted.

- Hold position for 20 seconds.
- Return to start and repeat with left leg.

E X E C U T I O N (both knees to chest)
- Gently pull both knees together toward your chest and hug them into your chest.
- Hold position for 20 seconds.

Stretch is felt along back and buttock.

Crossed-Legged Buttock Stretch

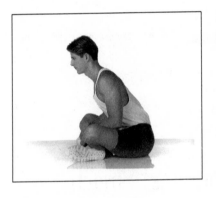

F O R M
- Sitting on the floor, cross the right leg in front of the left (Indian style). Knees will fall into a comfortable open position.
- Hands are resting on or in front of ankles.
- Keep abdominals contracted.

E X E C U T I O N
- Gently lean trunk forward.
- Hold position for 20 seconds.
- Return to start and repeat with the left leg.

Stretch is felt in each buttock.

Buttock/Hip Stretch (Iliotibial Band)

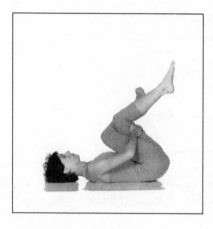

F O R M
- On your back, knees bent and feet flat on the floor.
- Cross the right knee over the left knee and bring both knees in toward chest.

E X E C U T I O N
- Wrap hands around legs and gently pull legs toward your chest and hold for 20 seconds.
- Return to start and repeat with opposite leg.

Stretch is felt on outside of each buttock.

Lower Back (Quadratus) Stretch

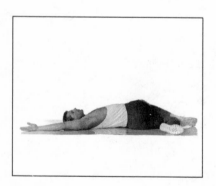

F O R M
- On your back, knees bent, feet flat on the floor.
- Drop both knees to the left side.

EXECUTION

- Slide the right upper leg over the left lower leg and extend it out.
- Extend right arm overhead with palm facing up.
- Hold for 20 seconds.
- Return to start and repeat on opposite side.

Stretch is felt in front of chest and along side of torso and outside of hip.

Hamstring Stretch

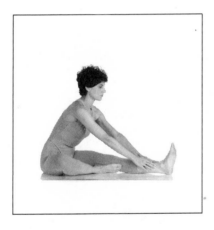

FORM

- Sit on the floor with back straight.
- Extend left leg straight out and place sole of right foot beside extended left thigh.

EXECUTION

- Slowly lean forward from your hips, keeping back straight.
- Stretch your hands out along your shin until you feel a stretch behind your knee.
- Hold the stretch for 20 seconds, then repeat on the other leg.

Seated Buttock Hip Stretch

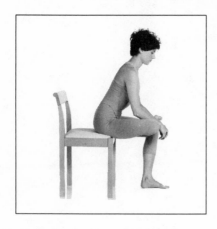

FORM
- Sit at the edge of a chair or table, keeping the left foot flat on the floor.
- Cross the right leg over the left, resting the ankle on the thigh just over the knee.
- Keep hands on the shin of your right leg.
- Keep your back straight.

EXECUTION
- Gently lean forward from the hips, keeping your back straight, until the stretch is felt at the side of the buttock.
- Hold position for 20 seconds.
- Return to the start position and repeat with the other leg.

Iliopsoas Stretch

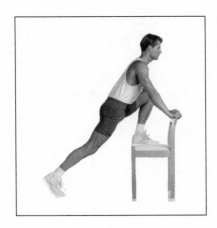

FORM
- Stand facing a low table or chair, toes straight ahead.
- Place left foot on table or chair, right leg extended fully behind you.

EXECUTION

- Lunge your hips forward, raising the heel of the standing leg and hold for 20 seconds.
- Return to start, repeat with opposite leg.
- Be sure to drop hip down toward table or chair and to maintain a straight back.

Stretch is felt in front of the hip of extended leg.

Calf Stretch

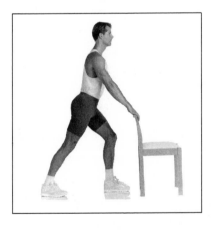

FORM

- Stand facing a wall, back of chair, or the like, with hands out for balance.
- Keep toes pointing straight ahead.
- Extend right leg behind you as far as possible, still keeping the heel on the floor.

EXECUTION

- Bend left knee only and lean slightly forward, keeping the knee directly over the toes; hold for 20 seconds.
- Return to start and repeat with left leg.

Stretch is felt in back of lower leg.

Quadriceps Stretch

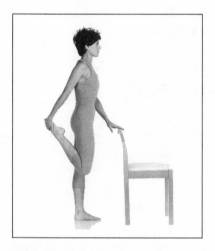

F O R M

- Stand facing back of chair or a wall.
- With the left hand holding on for balance and support, bend the right knee and grasp the foot behind you.

E X E C U T I O N

- Pull heel upward toward the buttock and hold for 20 seconds.
- Return to start and repeat with opposite leg.
- Tips: Contract your abdominals to keep your back from arching and don't lean forward.

Stretch is felt in front of thigh.

6

The Buttock Program
with Weights

For a greater challenge and for greater strength, endurance, and muscle tone, the next step in physical conditioning is weight training. This can involve various types of equipment—elastic bands, free weights, and/or weight machines. We recommend the use of free weights in the form of adjustable velcro-strapped weights and hand-held dumbbells. The velcro weight can vary its load using metal inserts. These usually range from 1 to 5 pounds or 5 to 10 pounds and can be strapped around the ankle or thigh. After successfully completing the advanced level of our nonweighted buttock program, you should be ready to add weights. The most important consideration when choosing what size weight to use is that proper form and technique must be maintained when executing the exercise. If you start exhibiting any of the don'ts listed among the pointers, the weight is too heavy. If you feel strain in any of your joints, your hips, knees, ankles, or low back, decrease the weight and possibly the number of reps and sets.

As in our nonweighted buttock program, use a maximum of 3–4 sets with 10–12 repetitions, and rest periods of 30–90 seconds. The training is in 3-week intervals with workouts 3 times a week. At the end of the third week, increase the weight and decrease reps and sets to that of week 1. Of course, if it takes longer to achieve higher reps and sets, continue until you are comfortable with the increasing weight. This program falls between the two extremes of strength and endurance training.

CHOOSING THE RIGHT WEIGHT

We recommend 1–1½-pound weights for beginner-level women and 2–2½ pounds for beginner-level men. Increase by 1–1½ and 2–2½ pounds respectively at the beginning of each of the next two levels, intermediate and advanced. The higher up the weights are placed on the leg the easier the exercise will be at that weight. Beginners should place weights on thighs and then progress to the ankles.

Maximum goals will be reached if your training is done on a regular basis and it varies in reps and sets, has progressive resistance (increases in weight), and includes stretching, aerobic activity, and proper rest and nutrition.

AVOID MUSCLE OR JOINT INJURY

To avoid or minimize the occurrence of muscle or joint injury when adding weights to your program, remember the following:
1. Increase training intensity gradually—do not add too much too soon.
2. Maintain good form.
3. Stretch before and after workouts.
4. Get adequate rest between workouts.
5. Eat properly.
6. Consult a doctor if you feel any persistent discomfort.